THE CAREER RESOURCE LIBRARY

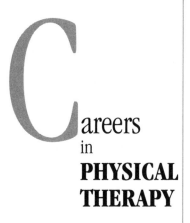

Careers
in
PHYSICAL
THERAPY

Trisha Hawkins

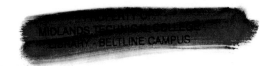

The Rosen Publishing Group, Inc.
NEW YORK

Published in 2001 by The Rosen Publishing Group, Inc.
29 East 21st Street, New York, NY 10010

Copyright © 2001 by Trisha Hawkins

First Edition

Cover photo © Richard T. Nowitz/Corbis

Library of Congress Cataloging-in-Publication Data

Hawkins, Trisha.
Careers in physical therapy / by Trisha Hawkins. — 1st ed.
p. ; cm. — (The career resource library)
Includes bibliographical references and index.
ISBN 0-8239-3192-7 (library binding)
1. Physical therapy—Vocational guidance. 2. Physical therapy assistants—Vocational guidance. [1. Physical therapy—Vocational guidance. 2. Vocational guidance.]
[DNLM: 1. Physical Therapy—Popular Works. 2. Vocational Guidance—Popular Works. WB 460 H394c 2001] I. Title. II. Series.
RM705 .H39 2001
615.8'2'023—dc21

2001001788

Manufactured in the United States of America

Contents

Introduction

Today, people are more active than ever. Everywhere you look, people are sweating in aerobics classes, jogging through parks, even tempting fate by practicing extreme sports. Physical activity isn't just child's play anymore: Adults are dancing, swimming, and jogging well into their seventies. It seems we can't sit still.

But not everyone is so active. Children are born with defects that impede their development. As adults age, they must cope with decreased physical function. Accident victims are bedridden, and athletes break bones and tear muscles and ligaments.

Physical therapists are needed to treat all of these afflictions. Known as PTs, they are trained to restore their patients' function to the highest possible level. PTs work in close partnership with their patients. Using methods like therapeutic exercise and hands-on techniques, and aided by physical therapist assistants (PTAs), they help individuals achieve their "personal best," whether that means regaining enough strength to walk across the room, restoring muscle function after a stroke or spinal cord injury, or building the necessary skills to become an Olympic athlete.

PTs work in a variety of health care settings. Some wear white coats; most work in casual street attire. As students, they gain experience by doing clinical trainings in hospitals, rehabilitation centers, nursing homes, or outpatient clinics. Later, they choose the setting where they want to work. Sometimes PTs open their own private offices or work through health agencies, treating people in their own homes. They may focus their practice on a certain group of people: children, older adults, athletes, or women, for example Each career in physical therapy is unique and built on a combination of factors: where the PT works and with which age group, what special skills the PT has acquired, and what health challenges he or she is really interested in and drawn to.

The History of Physical Therapy

The modern-day profession of physical therapy is the product of war and epidemic disease, and was born out of sheer necessity. There simply weren't enough doctors to care for all the wounded soldiers and polio victims at the start of the twentieth century. During World War I, the first physical therapy training programs were hastily put together. The new trainees joined with those who had experience treating the victims of polio to become the pioneers of a new profession.

The early practitioners of physical therapy were called reconstruction aides, and they worked in special reconstruction hospitals. Mary McMillan, who had received her training in physical therapy in England before World War I began and who helped train many of the new aides, is known as the first American physical therapist.

The American Physical Therapy Association (APTA)

After World War I ended in 1918, members of the newly born physical therapy profession—all of them women—struggled to find a place in peacetime America. Doctors and society as a whole did not yet realize how much they needed the services of these dedicated individuals and expected the former reconstruction aides to go back to whatever they had been doing before the war.

But the women took action; they were determined to establish physical therapy as a profession. In 1921, they formed the American Women's Physical Therapeutic Association. By the 1930s, the association had 1,000 members. Men also had begun to join the organization, which by then had changed its name to the American Physiotherapy Association.

In the 1940s and 1950s, PTs were very much in demand. Soldiers wounded in World War II needed competent, professional physical therapy, and the battles against the continuing polio epidemics that sickened and disabled children and adults were another kind of war for America, one in which PTs proved anew how much they were needed.

Today, the American Physical Therapy Association (APTA), as it is now called, has 75,000 members. There are 200 accredited university programs for PTs and 120,000 licensed PTs, including members and non-members of the APTA.

In Canada, the professional PT organization is called the Canadian Physiotherapy Association, and it has 9,000 members. Overall, there are 13,000 licensed PTs in Canada today, and thirteen universities where physiotherapists receive their training. PTs, PTAs, and students of physical therapy are all eligible to join the association. Members and nonmembers alike benefit from the association's advocacy and standard-setting for the profession.

Choosing a Career in Physical Therapy

The best way to determine if a career is for you is to learn as much about it as possible. PTs and PTAs work behind the scenes and one-on-one, so unless you or someone you are close to is injured or has a condition that requires physical therapy, you may not realize what a growing, wide-ranging, and important field it is.

Choosing a career is something that should not be taken lightly, and that is especially true if you are considering a career in health care. Based on interviews with dedicated PTs and PTAs, this book aims to give you insight into the profession of physical therapy. You'll read firsthand experiences from PTs and PTAs and find information about jobs, specialties, schooling, and things you can do now to prepare for a career in physical therapy.

A Career in
Physical Therapy

Physical therapists (PTs) are the heirs to the ancient tradition of healing by physical methods. At the same time, they are modern health professionals—highly skilled, educated, and trained to evaluate and treat health and movement problems that result from injury and disease, as well as disorders present at birth.

Choosing a career in physical therapy is a commitment to help people regain, improve, or maintain their ability to move and function in the world. There is no one standard of movement ability that everyone must reach. What's physically easy for one person may be a tremendous challenge for another.

Physical therapists are not physicians, although they work in conjunction with them. PTs do not prescribe medicine, and they do not perform surgery. Their hands-on methods—which include exercise, massage, mobilization, and the use of physical agents such as heat, cold, water, and electricity—are designed to reduce pain and improve an individual's ability to function in his or her world, whether that world is a playroom, kitchen, factory, concert hall, nursing home, or basketball court.

Physicians see people at crisis points; they perform operations or break the news when a test reveals that a person has a serious illness. Physical therapists, on the other hand, work one-on-one with their patients over a period of time. Along with physical therapist assistants (PTAs), they are there when a person begins the quietly courageous and sometimes painful process of rebuilding strength and endurance after an operation, illness, or injury.

Eric

Eric Quan is a PT who originally wanted to be a doctor. The story of how he discovered physical therapy reveals a lot about the special nature of the profession.

In college, Eric was a premed major. He had decided to become an orthopedic physician (a doctor who treats muscles and bones) specializing in the treatment of sports injuries. During his junior year, all the premed students had to volunteer at the local hospital, but no orthopedic doctors were available to oversee an internship. Eric was sent to the physical therapy department instead.

> When I walked in the first day, I saw people doing things I'd never seen before, having a great time, helping people. My first day there changed my whole outlook. I knew there was such a thing as physical therapy, but I thought it was just exercises a doctor prescribed for

you to do at home. I never knew there were actual people involved, I never knew there were physical therapists!

For six months, Eric observed physical therapists working with stroke patients, amputees, and all kinds of patients with all kinds of physical problems. He also helped set up equipment, cleaned up, and did general administrative work. He enjoyed it so much that after the internship ended, he asked if he could stay on for another six months. At the end of that time, Eric remembers, he chose to drop out of the premed program.

I knew I didn't want to do medicine. The interaction between the patient and the doctor is so different than it is between the patient and the PT. As a PT, you're with patients on the good days and the bad days, not like a doctor, who sees them one day and tells them, "Go to physical therapy and come back and see me in about one month's time." The doctors are seeing point A and then just jumping to point C— they never see point B.

The B part is what I really fell in love with: seeing patients daily, or at least a few times a week, having them tell me, "I've got pain," and then at the end of the session they're walking out with less pain or pain free. Of course, sometimes you can't fix it, but you try. My work gives me such an appreciation for the human body, how it restores itself, and how it deals with diseases and injuries.

Caring and Listening

If you choose to work in the field of physical therapy, you will be helping people meet their personal challenges, which, even though they are physical in nature, are also inner challenges. Over and over, the professionals who were interviewed for this book used words like "caring" and "listening." Listening is particularly important because if you don't listen, you may not understand what is wrong and why a person has come to you for help in the first place; you can't solve a problem until you know its exact nature. You won't be listening to just a list of symptoms and complaints; you'll be listening to hear what patients' physical goals are and what is most important to them in their lives.

As a medically trained helper and an attentive listener, your understanding and caring may help to ease emotional as well as physical pain. A PT may be there when an athlete realizes that despite all the effort, certain joints may never be stable and strong again. A PTA may be there when an old man with arthritic hands can't hold his coffee cup and has to take a minute to cry. PTs and PTAs see much triumph, but they also witness scenes of frustration and grief; after much hard work, some people have to accept that they have certain physical limitations or physical pain and that they must somehow learn to manage. Even then, people's will to live on and do the best they can may prove deeply inspiring.

Knowing Your Stuff

Even though PTs may lead with their human side, they are thoroughly trained medical professionals, working according to scientific principles. As a PT, you have to understand a certain body of knowledge and how to apply it. Working in a clinic without understanding what you are doing and why you are doing it is useless. On the other hand, constantly theorizing and studying and never applying your knowledge doesn't work either. You need the whole cycle of practice, in which knowledge and experience feed each other.

As more information comes to light about the human body and how it moves and functions, the educational and intellectual requirements for physical therapists and physical therapist assistants are becoming more rigorous. PTs must complete a master's degree, which takes two to three years if you already have a college degree, or six to seven years if you enter the program straight from high school. Physical therapy programs at some colleges and universities have initiated a doctoral program for PTs. PTAs must earn an associate's degree, which takes two years of study at a community or junior college.

Teaching

As a PT or PTA, you will be a teacher sometimes. You will teach your patients many physical skills and will instruct them as they exercise and learn how to take care of themselves. As you gain more experience, chances are you will also do some clinical teaching, passing on your skills to students and younger, less-experienced coworkers.

Helping People Move 2

Movement is basic to human life; it is almost as essential as eating, sleeping, and breathing. If you were very sick and were unable to move or get any exercise for more than about three weeks, your muscles and internal organs, such as your lungs and heart, would start to waste away.

Most of us take our ability to move for granted; we get up, sit down, walk, bend down, and reach out. We use our bodies to accomplish such everyday tasks as shopping, cooking, or getting to the bus stop, and we never give movement a second thought. We depend on our strength, endurance, and coordination at work, whether we load trucks or work at a computer. When we dance, run, jump, rock a baby in our arms, or hug somebody we're crazy about, we move for the sheer joy of it.

We may participate in a sport, acquiring special movement skills, working as a member of a team, and entering into competition. A few of us have special physical gifts and train for careers as professional athletes. Others become professional dancers, turning physical movement into an art form. Movement is at the center of our everyday lives. It is what allows us to function; it can also be a source of comfort, pleasure, and accomplishment.

This ability to move should not be taken for granted. A simple fact about being alive is that our bodies are vulnerable to disease, injury, and aging. We don't like to think about it until we have to, but the level of our physical fitness and our ability to function—to do the things we want to do—are subject to change. A battle with an illness, even if we get better, can leave our bodies weak. If we exercise or play sports, our drive to do better, get stronger, or play harder can backfire; we may overuse or misuse our bodies and suffer injury as a consequence.

Some babies and kids must cope with diseases or birth defects that make movement difficult, and even the healthiest adults must face the physical limitations that can come with old age. Accidents happen: car wrecks, fires, and falls. Stress, emotional difficulties, and habitual poor posture can create imbalance and pain in the body. When our ability to move is threatened, when our bodies hurt and are incapable of doing what we want them to do, that is the time when we become aware of our physical selves in earnest and start to appreciate what we have—at least temporarily—lost.

At times like these, physical therapy can help. PTs and PTAs treat people of all ages and backgrounds. Their patients have a wide variety of health concerns—some are healthy individuals who may have twisted an ankle or strained a shoulder; some are dancers and athletes whose livelihood depends on keeping their bodies healthy and injury free; others may be seriously ill or disabled.

Physical Methods

Newborn or aging, boxer or bookworm, able or disabled, energetic or slow-moving, people are physical creatures. The basic skills that allow people to move include:

- **Strength.** How much weight the muscles can lift, push, and pull.

- **Endurance.** Staying power; how long a person can keep doing an activity without tiring or overstressing muscles, bones, heart, and lungs.

- **Flexibility.** How limber a person is; what range of movement is possible; how smoothly the joints of the spine, shoulder, knee, ankle, wrist, fingers, elbow, foot, and jaw are able to move.

- **Coordination.** How well all the parts of the body work together to perform an action; how much the body is in sync with the brain.

- **Balance.** How steady and sure-footed a person is as he or she moves through space.

- **Agility.** How easily a person can switch the direction and speed of movement; how quickly someone can change his or her mind while moving; how he or she can swerve or jump.

It's easy to see that athletes and dancers possess these skills, but everybody depends on having at least a little bit of each one.

The methods that physical therapists and their assistants use to help people are physical, too, and include therapeutic exercise, functional training, and hands-on techniques.

Therapeutic Exercise

If you asked several PTs and PTAs to list their methods of treatment, therapeutic exercise—exercise that is individually prescribed and designed to heal—would probably be at the top of most lists. Even orthopedic physicians, whose job is to treat with surgery, would agree that therapeutic exercise may make some surgeries unnecessary and that, if surgery is required, exercise in the weeks or months following an operation is essential for regaining necessary body functions. A specific, individualized program of exercise can improve many different aspects of a person's movement ability.

Different types of exercise can improve different movement skills. When prescribing exercise, it is important to consider a person's age, physical condition, and temperament, what the person's personal movement goals are, what the person really is eager to get back to, and with what limitations the person can, or must, live.

Functional Training

The word "function" is all-important in physical therapy. It means the ability to do what needs to be done, whether it's hanging up your clothes or running from third base to home plate. To function doesn't necessarily mean that you do the thing you do speedily, with perfect grace, or even painlessly, but simply that you get it done. Three examples are an eighty-five-year-old woman who practices getting out of bed slowly and steadily, a worker on an assembly line who practices how to do his job more easily and safely, and a tennis player who practices her serve to maximize power and minimize strain. PTs and PTAs show people how to practice and offer hands-on help, as well as steadfast encouragement.

Hands-On Techniques

Other physical methods used by PTs and PTAs include numerous hands-on techniques. For example, a PTA may massage a painful back or use his or her hands to increase the range of movement of a frozen shoulder. Certain appliances, known as modalities, are also used. For more about these techniques, see chapter 7.

Rehabilitation

3

Understanding the concept of rehabilitation is important because it is at the heart of physical therapy. During World War I (1914–1918), wounded soldiers were cared for in what were known as reconstruction hospitals. During World War II (1939–1945), reconstruction gave way to rehabilitation.

The word "reconstruction" brings to mind a mechanical process, like putting something together again after it has been broken, but the newer word, "rehabilitation," is derived from the Latin words *habilitare* and *habilitas*, which mean "to enable" and "ability," combined with the prefix "re," which means "again." As the new goal of physical therapy, rehabilitation came to mean not just mending an injury but increasing a wounded soldier's ability to regain his function, spirit, and ability to live his life fully.

Howard A. Rusk, who served as a doctor in the air force during World War II, played a major role in developing the concept of rehabilitation. In his autobiography, *A World to Care For*, Dr. Rusk describes seeing the wounded soldiers who were flown in from the front: "boys with burns, and half their faces blown away, without arms or legs, boys with broken backs."

Dr. Rusk's job was to treat these soldiers and send as many of them as possible back to active duty, but his concern was far beyond merely patching them up. He wanted to provide these young men, many of whom were paraplegics (paralyzed from the waist down), with the best treatment and the best chance of becoming active again, holding jobs, having fun, and making a contribution to society. Another quote from Dr. Rusk's book shows how much programs of rehabilitation were needed, both for the soldiers and for the rest of the population.

> I recall someone asking me how paraplegics had lived up to that time. The answer was, except in extremely rare cases, they usually died—their life expectancy in those days was often less than a year. They got terrible bedsores, developed kidney and bladder problems, and simply lay in bed, waiting for death. It was almost the same with strokes. The old wives' tale was that you had one stroke, and then you sat around waiting for a second one, or a third one, or however many it took to kill you. If you had any kind of brain injury affecting your locomotive functions, everyone assumed your life was finished.

With the help of Dr. George G. Deaver, Dr. Rusk set up a school to train people to work with the injured and disabled in an active, comprehensive way. Some of these people became physical therapists, and others were doctors who would soon establish the specialty of physical medicine. Today, these doctors are known as physiatrists—doctors of rehabilitation and physical medicine, who often work side by side with physical therapists.

Joan

Joan Edelstein, a PT who is now director of the physical therapy program at Columbia University, met Dr. Rusk when she was a teenager. Inspired by her meetings with Rusk and with Dr. Henry Kessler, another rehabilitation pioneer, Joan decided to study physical therapy and work in the field of rehabilitation, which she defines as:

> The branch of health care that endeavors to restore a patient to his maximum functional capacity. Rehabilitation emphasizes function in the sense of returning to work, returning to school, or returning to leisure activities—whatever the person cares to do.

Joan studied at New York University (NYU) and landed her first job at what is now the Rusk Institute, in New York City, which pioneered the team approach to rehabilitation. Joan and two other PTs worked in the children's division, along with physicians, occupational therapists, and speech therapists. Most of the kids had cerebral palsy and had trouble coordinating their muscles; some had had amputations; others had a condition called spina bifida, which means that at birth, a part of the spinal cord is left exposed, often paralyzing the child's body beneath the level at which the spinal cord is exposed.

17

When asked what it was like to work with her young patients as part of a rehabilitation team, Joan offers an example of a three-year-old boy, referred for treatment because he has spina bifida. The boy's parents would of course be very concerned—their son has probably had medical treatment from the day he was born. By the age of three, Joan says, the concern will be how the child is going to move around and manage in preschool, then in kindergarten and up through the grades. A program of rehabilitation can help such a child engage in many activities.

Today, the process of rehabilitation happens not only in special rehabilitation hospitals and centers, but in all the different places where PTs choose to practice: schools, regular hospitals, outpatient clinics, nursing facilities, private homes and offices, community health centers, and industrial and corporate settings.

Sometimes, as at the Rusk Institute, rehabilitation requires a team approach, but the process can also be a simple one-on-one partnership between a PT and a patient. It all depends on the patient and the nature of the health problem, or problems, with which he or she is faced.

The Future: Prevention

The basic concepts of rehabilitation—that you can "come back" from injury and disease; that the whole person, not just the disease or injury, needs to be cared for; and that even if you remain severely disabled, you can find ways to live and thrive—continue to inspire health care professionals and patients alike.

As the benefits of therapeutic exercise and hands-on techniques have become widely known, the principles of rehabilitation have been extended to include the principles of prevention. This is a rediscovery of something that doctors in ancient Greece promoted. Their idea was that exercise is good for your health and that insufficient exercise can be detrimental to overall bodily functioning. Herodicus, who lived in the fourth century BC and was a wrestler as well as a doctor, said it is "just as important to provide against diseases in the healthy man as to cure him who is already attacked."

Today, we are realizing that many conditions can be prevented by exercise and functional training and education, and that good health can be preserved by those same methods. These ideas have opened up many new jobs in physical therapy.

Prevention, an ancient yet newly rediscovered idea, emphasizes health and wellness. A health care professional such as a PT can sometimes nip health problems in the bud. With a PT's expert advice, people can use exercise and other methods to increase their wellness, strengthen their hearts, deepen their breathing, keep their bones healthy and their minds sharp, and nourish their immune systems. For example, health issues particular to women, such as those pertaining to their reproductive systems, were long considered something women could only accept and suffer through. Now PTs are setting up health and wellness practices that address women's health concerns with an emphasis on prevention.

Holistic Health

As more and more people search for ways to promote health and wellness, many have been drawn to the idea of holistic health. According to the dictionary, holistic means "emphasizing the importance of the whole, and the interdependence of its parts." Holistic medicine treats the whole person, somewhat like Dr. Rusk did when he rehabilitated soldiers during World War II, but today the focus is on wellness and prevention as well.

One problem with holistic practice, however, is that it is a wide-open field with few real standards. It's sometimes hard for people to figure out who is qualified and what kind of therapy, treatment, or learning experience might really be beneficial. Many PTs make use of complementary therapies in their practices and advise their patients on matters such as nutrition, that is, how your diet can play a role in improving health and preventing disease. In Canada, many PTs are trained to give acupuncture treatments, which are an accepted part of physical therapy in that country.

No one can predict the future, but it seems that PTs—who use physical, noninvasive methods, who are educated in scientific principles, and who know the importance of a caring attitude—are already becoming leaders in the fields of prevention and wellness.

What Is a
Physical Therapist?

4

The American Physical Therapy Association (APTA) has come up with a streamlined definition of a physical therapist. According to the APTA, PTs are "health care professionals who evaluate and treat health problems resulting from injury and disease."

In this chapter, we'll begin to take this definition apart and look at it piece by piece to get a better understanding of who works in physical therapy and what that work really involves.

"Health Problems Resulting from Injury and Disease"

Which injuries and diseases are helped by physical therapy? To mention every single one would take pages, but here is the APTA's list of the most common reasons why people receive physical therapy:

- Lower back pain
- Neck pain

- Shoulder, arm, wrist, or hand problems
- Knee, ankle, or foot problems
- Carpal tunnel syndrome (pain and weakness in the hand from repetitive motion)
- Sprains and muscle strains
- Arthritis
- Cardiac (heart) rehabilitation
- Rehabilitation after a serious injury or disease
- Chronic respiratory (breathing) problems
- Stroke rehabilitation
- Problems with balance
- Disabilities in newborns
- Prenatal and postnatal problems
- Hip fractures
- Incontinence (involuntary urination)
- Fitness and wellness needs

PTs and PTAs are trained as generalists, which means that they are qualified to work with patients who have any of the health issues listed above. In practice, though, each of these health care problems can become a specialty, and it is only with experience and sometimes further clinical study that a clinician becomes expert in one of more of these areas.

Let's go back to the APTA's definition and look at the very first part of the sentence.

"Health Care"

Physical therapy is provided in a number of health care settings. About 30 percent of PTs are employed by hospitals. The other 70 percent work in private physical therapy offices, sports facilities, rehabilitation centers, outpatient clinics, schools, nursing homes, corporate and industrial health centers, and in people's homes. Some PTs also teach in universities that offer degrees in physical therapy.

Let's move on to the next word in the APTA's definition.

"Professionals"

PTs are health care professionals. PTAs, on the other hand, are not, strictly speaking, professionals. They do provide physical therapy, but they are paraprofessionals—PTAs assist PTs in the same way that a paralegal might assist a lawyer.

What makes a physical therapist a professional? Here are a few of the things that are used to define a professional.

- As a member of a profession, you are a member of a group of people who are your peers, or colleagues, and who share your devotion to a certain kind of work. Each profession has its own association, an organization that sets educational and practice standards. The professional association for physical therapists in the United States is the American Physical Therapy Association. In Canada, the association is the Canadian Physiotherapy Association. In today's rather competitive health care marketplace, the associations promote and advocate for the profession. The associations also try to attract capable people to the profession. For instance, the APTA has programs to increase the number of Hispanic and African American people in the profession of physical therapy.

• Professionals are specially educated and trained to do what they do. Physical therapists must complete a master's degree. Some universities offer an entry-level doctoral degree. For more about education, see chapter 8. Like physicians and lawyers, PTs must pass a national examination and be licensed in the state in which they practice.

• Professionals often command a higher salary than people who are not as extensively educated or who are not qualified to assume as much responsibility. According to the APTA, the median yearly salary for a physical therapist is $55,000; that means that half of the salaries are below that level and half are above. A PT's salary depends on position, years of experience, degree of education, geographic location, and practice setting. Some physical therapists earn $100,000 a year or more.

• Often, a professional will supervise others. PTs supervise and are helped by two groups of people: PTAs and physical therapy aides, which are discussed in chapter 6.

• A professional has a specialized body of knowledge and functions independently and responsibly within his or her area of expertise. A PT may or may not work under a physician's referral but does make many decisions. The APTA's definition states that PTs "evaluate and treat." That means they decide what needs doing and how to do it.

Helpful Character Traits

The human qualities of empathy and compassion are necessities for a career in physical therapy. The dictionary defines empathy as "identification with and understanding of another's situation, feelings, and motives." Compassion is being aware of—and wanting to relieve—the suffering of others.

Other helpful qualities are patience, creativity, calmness, a sense of humor, and a complete lack of prejudice. It is essential to have the ability to think, to reflect, to make decisions, and to problem-solve. Good communication skills and self-confidence are also necessary: You'll be standing up for what you think is right for your patient as you work alongside physicians, nurses, and other types of therapists, as well as communicating with your patients and their families. Physical therapist Margaret Plack says, "You have to be able to make therapy fun, and be very much a caring person. You've got to be a person who really wants to know people and learn what is most important to them . . . it's very much a relationship."

Evaluating the Patient

The most active words in the APTA's definition of a PT—the verbs that really get to the nitty-gritty of what PTs do—are "evaluate and treat." These are the actions that a PT performs day in and day out. No matter where PTs work or what problems they are helping their patients to overcome, individualized evaluation and treatment are what every PT does with each patient. We will discuss treatment in chapter 7.

To evaluate means "to determine the condition by careful study." To solve a problem, you first have to know what the problem is in full detail. The first things a PT does when he or she sees a new patient are take a full medical history, examine the patient, and administer appropriate tests. From the information gathered by the PT, he or she is able to make a detailed evaluation, or assessment.

A PT uses many skills and qualities during an evaluation: respect and caring for the patient, intelligence, sensitivity, scientific and clinical knowledge, and experience, as well as the ability to listen to the patient's story. During the physical examination, the PT palpates, or touches, the patient's muscles, bones, tendons, ligaments, joints, and skin.

After learning as much about the patient as possible, the PT uses his or her intelligence, scientific knowledge, clinical training, experience, common sense, and human understanding to create a treatment plan. (This is the job of the physical therapist—PTAs and aides do not have the training or the legal right to evaluate patients or create a treatment plan.)

What follows is a general outline of the patient evaluation process:

- **Take a medical/personal history.** Even though a PT has the patient's medical records and can refer to them, he or she will want to listen to the patient describe his or her aches and pains, when the symptoms started, and how those symptoms have affected the patient's life. The PT will want to know what the patient's living situation is, what responsibilities the patient is dealing with, and any other factors that affect the patient's life and health. It's important that he or she listen to the unspoken messages the patient may be sending, as well as the words that are spoken. The PT may also talk with members of the patient's family. Later, family members may need to learn how to assist in their loved one's recovery.

- **Evaluate strength.** The PT will measure and evaluate the patient's strength. Machines have been designed to do this, but usually a PT uses his or her hands to see how forcefully patients can push against them with their own hands, their shoulder, or their lower leg. The evaluation of strength gives the PT and the patient a place to start so that future progress can be measured.

- **Evaluate ROM.** The PT may measure the range of motion, or ROM, of his or her patient's joints. Does the joint have its full movement, or does pain and stiffness limit its range of motion? What range of movement in a joint is possible when the patient actively moves his or her own arm or leg? What ROM is possible when the patient allows the PT to move the arm or leg? Here's where the sensitivity of a physical therapist's hands comes into the picture. In the case of a patient with arthritis, for example, which is a disease that causes the joints to become stiff, damaged, or inflamed, the PT will use his or her hands to move and probe the patient's affected joints to determine the nature of the damage the arthritis may have caused. Sometimes a device called a goniometer is used to measure the ROM of a joint. A goniometer is a protractor with long arms; it can measure the exact number of degrees a joint can move.

- **Evaluate a patient's pain.** If the patient suffers from pain, the PT will ask where the pain is located, when it occurs, and how severe it is. Margaret Plack, who worked for many years at a school for kids and adults with cerebral palsy and other developmental problems, stresses the importance of building a relationship and communicating with a patient. This is important because the patient's degree of pain may make him or her reluctant to be touched.

- **Evaluating function.** This may be the most basic part of the evaluation process. The PT may ask his or her patient to perform simple actions, such as getting up from a chair, walking across the room, or reaching out to open a door. The PT will want to know what kind of life activities the patient is involved in and may ask the patient to demonstrate how he or she performs these everyday activities and tasks. Later the PT may be able to teach his or her patient new ways of moving that make certain tasks less painful, safer, or easier to accomplish.

- **Other evaluations.** Evaluations may also be done on a person's posture, gait (how he or she walks), and skin condition. Other types of tests include cardiopulmonary (how the patient breathes and how well his or her heart is functioning), neurological (how well the brain and nervous system are working), and sensory (which could involve an action as simple as brushing something lightly across the skin of a patient's forearm).

The Importance of the PT's Evaluation Skills

In some states, a physician sends a patient to a PT by means of a referral, or prescription. In other states, patients can go directly to a PT for treatment without having to get a referral from a physician; this is known as direct access. In Canada, people in all the provinces can choose to go directly to a PT, but some insurance plans in that country still require a doctor's prescription before they will cover charges for physiotherapy visits.

When a patient comes directly to a physical therapist without first seeing a physician for an examination and diagnosis, that PT's evaluation skills need to be especially strong. In those cases, the PT decides the nature of the patient's problem and whether it is something that the PT can treat.

Another situation in which evaluation skills are crucial is when a PT is treating someone whose condition or source of pain has not yet been pinpointed. Sometimes PTs see patients who have many-layered problems that contribute to chronic pain (meaning that it lasts a long time or comes back again and again) and loss of function. In these cases, too, evaluation skills are very important.

On the other hand, PTs who work in hospitals are often working with people whose problems are quite clear and who have already been diagnosed and treated by a physician. In these cases, a PT's evaluation is not as crucial, although it is still extremely important. Without evaluation, a PT cannot create a meaningful plan of care.

Physical Therapist Assistants and Physical Therapy Aides

6

The APTA defines physical therapist assistants as "skilled health providers who work under the supervision of physical therapists." A physical therapist assistant, or PTA, is qualified to carry out most physical therapy treatments.

PTAs do not evaluate patients, they do not create a plan of care, and they cannot decide (though they can advise) whether a treatment plan is complete. PTAs work under the supervision of PTs, but that doesn't mean that the PT is looking over the PTA's shoulder all the time. What it usually means is that a PT is "under the same roof" and is available for consultation.

PTAs record the patient's responses to treatment and report to the PT on the outcome of each treatment. Because they may work more regularly with the patient than the PT, they see the patient's progress, inch by inch.

PTAs must complete an accredited, two-year education program, typically offered through a community or junior college. They graduate with an associate's degree. More than half of all states require PTAs to be licensed, registered, or certified. Different states have different rules. To find out what the rules are in your state, contact the Federation of State Boards of Physical Therapy at www.fsbpt.org.

Like PTs, PTAs work in many different kinds of settings. Many join the APTA and take continuing education courses to add to their expertise. The median yearly income for a physical therapist assistant is $30,000 a year.

Beebe

Beebe Haniff is a PTA who works in a large physical therapy clinic connected to a hospital. She came to the United States from Guyana, in South America. Back home, Beebe had taught grade school, and when she came to the States and enrolled in a community college, she had thought she would probably wind up teaching in her new country, too.

But then Beebe started investigating other departments and asking other students what they were majoring in. A lot of them said they were studying for a two-year associate's degree as a physical therapist assistant. Beebe started to do research on physical therapy in her community college library.

> I was interested because back home in Guyana I had never heard of physical therapy. I don't think we even had it there when I was a kid growing up—we're a third world country, and we're so poor. When a kid or anybody had a

problem, we usually picked some leaves from a special plant or bush and boiled up some tea for them. Going to the doctor was the last resort. When things got really bad—when you were close to dying—that's when you went to the doctor.

Beebe discovered that PTAs often work with older people recovering from strokes or suffering from painful arthritis in their joints. She knew she liked helping people, and she began to think that physical therapy might suit her better than teaching grade school.

Older people are so grateful when you do something for them. PTAs do a lot—we're the workhorses. We're paid less than the PTs, but we do a lot of the same work. It's a good job, but only if it's right for you. You've got to give so much of yourself, of your energy, especially when you're working with very sick people who need encouragement.

Sinclair

Sinclair Scott, a PTA and an athlete who works in a nursing home, was interviewed for the APTA pamphlet *Fit Teens,* which is also available online at the APTA Web site, www.apta.org. He says:

This is my calling. I treat senior citizens. I find it very rewarding to work with the elderly because I learn a lot about life from their experiences!

Some of my patients have a hard time feeling good about themselves. Much of the treatment involves getting to know them and helping them feel comfortable around me. I feel great when I can help people become independent and return home after they've had a stroke or fractured a hip, for instance.

When asked whether you can make a good living as a physical therapist assistant, Sinclair answers, "Yes, you can. But if you're in it for the money, you won't make it. You've got to care."

The Future for PTAs

If you are thinking about becoming a PTA, most of the material in this book about PTs applies to you, too. Just remember, as a PTA you will not evaluate patients or create a treatment plan. Another important thing to consider is that if you later decide that you want to qualify as a physical therapist, your PTA coursework will not transfer—it will not count toward a physical therapy degree. Of course, your schooling and experience as a PTA will help you in your studies and will be a good base for a career in physical therapy, but you will have to start from scratch on the academic side and earn your physical therapy degree.

In the late 1990s, many PTAs—especially those who worked in nursing homes—were let go or had to accept reduced hours. This was due to many factors, such as the Balanced Budget Act of 1997, insurance and Medicare/Medicaid cutbacks, and the fact that more and more schools are offering PTA training. PTs experienced some of the same problems, but PTAs were the hardest hit. As of 2001, the APTA planned to devote much time and effort to improving the job outlook for physical therapist assistants. PTs know how valuable, dependable, and dedicated PTAs are.

Physical Therapy Aides

Physical therapy aides work under the direct supervision of a PT or PTA. They keep the treatment area clean and organized and prepare the equipment. When patients need assistance moving to or from a treatment area, aides push them in a wheelchair or give them support. Part of an aide's job may be clerical work such as answering the phone and ordering supplies. Sometimes aides assist in treatments, but only as directed and only in the presence of a PT or PTA.

No special training is required to become a physical therapy aide. Aides earn approximately $20,000 a year. For some, a job as a physical therapy aide is an end in itself, but sometimes young people who are interested in becoming PTs or PTAs will work for a time as an aide.

Treating the Patient

7

After evaluating a patient, a PT devises a treatment plan based on the information gathered. The PT shares the outcome of the evaluation process with the patient and explains the proposed plan of care. If the patient agrees to the plan, the PT will begin to treat the patient, sometimes with the help of a PTA. As part of the plan of care, the PT and the patient will set short-term and long-term goals.

PTs and PTAs use numerous hands-on techniques, such as mobilization and massage, to treat patients. For example, a PT may massage a painful back or may use his or her hands to increase the range of movement of a shoulder. Sometimes exercise machines are part of the program. Often, though, a PT's most important tools are his or her hands.

PTs and PTAs also may use certain appliances, known as modalities, that employ water, heat, cold, and electricity to ease pain, undo tension, or stimulate muscles. For instance, a PTA may apply a hot pack to a tight shoulder or use a machine to stimulate an injured area with carefully controlled electric current.

There are many physical therapy treatment options available to PTs. In choosing which to use, a PT is exercising clinical skill. Knowing what not to do is every bit as important as knowing what to do. The following are some examples of methods and modalities.

Therapeutic Exercise

Exercise can be therapeutic. It is perhaps a physical therapist's most important tool—it is certainly the most widely used. Sometimes exercise is passive; for instance, if a person is unable to move a leg or an arm, a PT can exercise and stretch that limb to prevent the joint from becoming stiff and losing its range of motion. Exercise can also, of course, be active, which means that the patient is able to do it independently.

Sometimes a good home-exercise plan, with specific exercises written down for the patient, will be all that is needed for a speedy recovery. In some cases, a PT helps with certain movements. That is known as active-assisted exercise.

Exercise may be as basic as repeated lifting and lowering of a patient's leg to build up enough strength to begin walking. It may mean working out on a machine with weights to build strength or walking on a treadmill to build up endurance and cardiovascular health.

PTs may set up patients on different kinds of exercise machines that are designed to improve strength. They work with the patient—slowly increasing the resistance weight. They may also use a physioball, which is a big, colorful, plastic ball on which patients can sit or stretch.

Other types of exercise may involve doing very specific movements to increase the ROM of a specific joint or stretch a specific tendon. A PT, who knows from the evaluation where someone is weak or tight, how efficiently he or she can breathe, and how coordinated he or she is, can customize an exercise program for each patient.

The great thing about exercise is that most people eventually can do it independently; what they have learned from their PT can become part of their daily routines, something they can do for themselves.

Manual Therapy and Massage Therapy

The word "manual" comes from *manus*, the Latin word for "hand." Manual is defined as "done by the hands" and "employing human rather than mechanical energy." All PTs do some form of manual therapy, but some may really specialize in it. There are even national associations of manual therapists; one of these is the American Academy of Orthopaedic Manual Physical Therapists (AAOMPT).

PTs use skilled hand movements to mobilize or manipulate tissues and joints. Manual therapy is successful in managing pain, increasing ROM, reducing inflammation (swelling) or restriction, inducing relaxation, and improving pulmonary (breathing) function.

Hand movements can be slow or quick, and they can move parts of the patient's body a little or a lot. Manual therapy is a tool that is widely used in physical therapy because it is often effective in treating musculoskeletal problems like back, neck, or shoulder pain. Of all the physical therapy interventions, it is perhaps the one that is most truly both an art and a science.

Massage is a well-established manual technique in physical therapy. PTs and PTAs are qualified to do massage as part of physical therapy treatment. Massage can reduce pain, relax muscles, and increase circulation, and thus may help patients tolerate greater movement in their joints or enable them to exercise more safely and for a longer period of time.

Chris

Chris Barrett, a PT who uses manual therapy to treat many dancers and musicians, describes how she measures progress in manual therapy and how she works to make her patients able to move, function, and exercise on their own.

> One of the things I try to do in a manual therapy treatment session is to link my result to an objective "before and after" test. So I'll have my sequence of tests that I'll do for a specific joint or a specific motion.
>
> When people have low back and hip problems, we spend a lot of time trying to improve their walking because symmetrical (well-balanced) walking is very healthy for the joints and muscles, and asymmetrical (unbalanced) walking really causes wear and tear. So I have a couple of little motion tests I'll do, and then when I treat, I always try to do a test before and

a test after, partly to see if I made an objective difference, rather than just having the patient get off the table and asking them, "How do you feel?" Sometimes you change something and they don't feel it for a couple of days.

But the tests are partly for the patient, too, so they realize that I'm looking at an objective outcome and that it's not just a manual therapy. People get dependent on you. They start feeling that what is really getting them better is your hands on them. I feel like my putting my hands on them facilitates them moving better; it frees up their range of motion. But the fact that they are moving better, walking better, is what really improves their condition.

Other Therapies and Modalities

Pulmonary Therapy

To help a patient breathe better, PTs may perform special forms of massage, such as percussion and vibration. Pounding on the patient's back and creating a vibratory movement in the patient's chest clears secretions out of the lungs. PTs may also give a patient lessons in how to breathe more deeply and efficiently.

Hydrotherapy and Aquatherapy

Water can be a useful healing tool for a PT. Whirlpools can relieve pain, increase circulation, or cleanse an arm or leg after a cast or splint has been removed. Contrasting baths that alternate hot and cold water in a specific time sequence are used to treat arthritis of the hands and feet and speed recovery from injuries.

Sometimes PTs recommend that patients exercise in a pool. Water greatly reduces the weight of the patient's body by increasing buoyancy, thus making it possible to exercise with less pain and without harming the joints. The water temperature is kept at about 92 degrees Fahrenheit—warmer than recreational pools. Many types of therapeutic equipment can be used in the pools, such as lifts, steps, parallel bars, handrails, and special chairs.

During the first half of the twentieth century, pool therapy was used to help children and adults who were paralyzed by polio. Later, many pools were drained and paved over because they took up too much space. Recently, however, aquatherapy has made a comeback because it has proven to be beneficial to many patients who have arthritis or spinal cord injuries, or who are recovering from certain types of operations.

Cryotherapy and Heat Therapy

The use of cold, or cryotherapy, is widely used as a physical therapy treatment. Cold packs can reduce swelling and pain after musculoskeletal injuries.

Heat is used in many forms. Hot packs are pouches filled with silica gel. When they are warmed and placed on a part of a patient's body, they can relax muscles and improve circulation. The packs are kept in a tank, which contains water that is warmed to 160 degrees Fahrenheit. They are wrapped in layers of towels and are placed on the area to be treated for fifteen minutes. Often, a hot pack treatment will relax muscles to the point where the patient can tolerate more activity during the exercise part of the physical therapy session.

Electricity

Electrical current may also be used to reduce chronic pain and help heal wounds. Electricity can be used in many ways, such as electrical stimulation, when a PT uses a machine that sends electric current into an injured muscle. In another treatment, called iontophoresis, an electric current drives chemicals or medicines deep into injured body tissues to reduce inflammation.

Ultrasound

High frequency sound waves penetrate through tissue and can create a kind of deep heat to promote healing and reduce pain.

Assistive Devices, Prostheses, and Orthotics

PTs can help their patients select assistive devices, such as canes, walkers, or wheelchairs. They are also trained to teach people how to use these devices to help them function more easily and safely in their daily activities. People may need to learn a new way of walking in order to make the most of an assistive device. A PT can teach a person who has had a leg amputated to walk with a prosthesis, or artificial leg. A child or adult can be fitted with a brace, or orthotic, on an ankle, leg, back, or hand to stabilize and strengthen the area.

Complementary Therapies

Nontraditional therapies and techniques may be used by PTs to enhance or complete a more traditional course of physical therapy treatments. It is the decision of the individual PT which complementary therapies—if any—he or she chooses to train in and incorporate into his or her physical therapy practice. Complementary therapies include acupressure, Qigong, yoga, myofascial release, craniosacral therapy, Rolfing, Hellerwork, soma, Pilates, Alexander technique, Feldenkrais Awareness through Movement and Functional Integration, neuromuscular therapy, and reflexology. There is also acupuncture, which involves inserting needles, something that is beyond the scope of conventional physical therapy in the United States.

Each Treatment Plan Is Unique

As you can see, there is a wide range of physical therapy treatment options. Each patient is evaluated as an individual, and each treatment plan is unique. The challenge is knowing when to apply it, when to adapt it, and when to modify it to meet the needs of each individual. Every patient who has had a stroke doesn't get the same plan. What works for one stroke victim may not work for another. Other injuries and effects, as well as the patient's lifestyle, are factors in choosing a treatment plan. Someone who has children and an active job would get a much different plan than would an elderly, retired person.

Treatment plans are not written in stone. Evaluation is a continuing process, and the physical therapist—with the input of the PTA—is always aware of how the patient is progressing. The PT must be ready to reevaluate and change the treatment plan in response to how the patient is doing.

Physical Therapy as Teaching

Almost every physical therapist who was interviewed for this book stressed that perhaps the most important thing a PT or PTA does is teach. It's not the kind of teaching a schoolteacher does in a classroom, though, although some PTs do go on to become professors or provide clinical instruction for physical therapy students. Most of the teaching that PTs and PTAs do is one-on-one and practical—teaching people exercises to do at home, teaching them how to use assistive devices, and teaching them better ways to move and go about their daily activities.

Today, such education is more important than ever because patients' insurance usually will pay for only a certain number of visits to a PT. Sometimes the PT wishes that he or she could work with a patient for a longer time, but he or she must deal with the reality of the insurance system. It's up to the PT and PTA to educate their patients so that they can continue physical therapy independently and complete the recovery process. PTs also teach and educate patients' family members so they can help, too.

An Important Note About Insurance and Paperwork

During the evaluation and treatment process, PTs keep in contact with their patients' physicians and insurance companies, whether it be private insurance, Medicare, or Medicaid. PTs must keep accurate records of the evaluation and treatment process so they can show the physicians how each patient is progressing and justify the patient's physical therapy treatment to the insurance company. There is a great deal of paperwork that must be generated, and there is a lot of negotiating with insurance companies, trying to get them to cover the number of visits that a patient really requires.

These days, paperwork and health care are inseparable. The APTA helps its members cope with insurance frustrations by keeping them informed and continuing to lobby for adequate funding for physical therapy treatments.

Outcome

After the evaluation and treatment, there is an outcome—a result of all the work the patient and the PT and PTA have done. PTs and PTAs gain great satisfaction from their work because they are able to contribute so much to their patients' recovery. Of course, life is not a fairy tale, and recovery and rehabilitation are not always complete. Some patients require surgery, and nothing a PT does can change that. Physical therapy does not cure everything.

Sometimes, maintaining a patient's movement ability is in itself a kind of victory. For example, some people are able to recover much of their lost function after they have a stroke, but others are considered successes if they are simply able to stay at their current level. If they are walking, their goal is to continue walking and not regress. On the other hand, most patients are able to recover or improve, and PTs and PTAs have many inspiring stories to tell.

Alex

Alex Bagley, who works as a PT in a big-city hospital, tells about working with a man who had been operated on for cancer and wound up spending almost three months in the intensive care unit in the hospital.

Martin had spent three months in intensive care, so he got really debilitated [feeble]. After about three weeks, if you don't get patients going, they just spiral down. Not only your muscles, but your organ systems waste away if you're in bed. When I first met Martin, he was on a ventilator [a machine that helps you breathe], and I ended up getting him to use a walker, and he went off for further rehabilitation.

His last day in the hospital, I walked him without the walker, holding his arm, giving him support, but basically he was doing it all on his own. He said, "This is the best graduation present." And I said, "You know, Martin, I just felt like today I wanted to show you that you were really going to make it." It gave me such a charge—this guy really, really appreciated the fact that he had been shown that he was coming back; that he was going to walk again.

Getting Started: Preparation, Education, and Training

8

People take all kinds of routes to a career in physical therapy. Your story will be unique.

Tracy

Tracy Sawyer's sister had been in an accident and had had multiple surgeries on her knee. After the operations, she entered a program of physical therapy. Around that same time, Tracy saw the movie *The Other Side of the Mountain*, which was about a famous skier who went through physical therapy after she had an accident and became paralyzed. The movie was a tremendous inspiration to Tracy. By the time she finished junior high school, she was sure she wanted to be a physical therapist, and she particularly wanted to work with accident victims and people with spinal cord injuries.

Tracy volunteered at a local hospital during high school and went on to earn a degree in physical therapy. She later worked for twelve years in a special hospital where she treated many people who had serious spinal cord injuries. Every day, she says, she learned something new.

What You Can Do Now

If you're intrigued by the idea of a career in physical therapy, one of the first things you should do is to find a way to observe real PTs in action. Chances are you'll be able to find a hospital, nursing home, rehabilitation center, outpatient clinic, or private practice where you will be allowed to volunteer or observe.

Observation time in any type of health care setting will be informative. If you find a place to observe that seems interesting and right, the experience can teach you a lot about the profession and how you might eventually become part of it.

Summers are a good time to get experience, too. The American Sports Medicine Institute in Birmingham, Alabama, offers a summer camp for people ages twelve to eighteen that offers a look into musculoskeletal surgery, athletic training, physical therapy, and prevention of athletic injuries. Maybe there are similar programs in your area.

Of course, after seeing it up close, you may decide that a career in physical therapy isn't for you after all. That's a valuable step, too, because it frees you to explore other career options; maybe there is another job in the health care field that is a better fit for you. Find a way to put yourself in a position in which you can be exposed to the clinical nuts and bolts of a physical therapy practice, and then trust your instincts about whether it's the career for you.

High School Classes

Another absolutely essential thing to do as you prepare for a career in physical therapy is to study. Getting into a physical therapy program is competitive—getting good grades, especially in your science courses, is your best shot at being accepted into an entry-level master's degree program. High school courses in biology, chemistry (which serves as a basis for the study of physiology), and physics (which will help you understand the physical laws of the body and movement) will give you a good grounding in the sciences and will help prepare you for the science that will be the academic foundation of your education once you get into graduate school, including the following:

- **Anatomy.** For physical therapy students, the study of anatomy involves, among other things, an in-depth study of the musculoskeletal system—each bone, muscle, ligament, and tendon has a specific location, purpose, and name. Neuroanatomy is the study of the structure and function of the brain, the spinal cord, and the nerves.

- **Physiology.** The study of how the systems and organs of the body function and influence each other. Systems of the body of particular importance in physical therapy include the digestive, circulatory, nervous, cardiopulmonary, musculoskeletal, and immune systems.

- **Kinesiology.** The study of movement: how the musculoskeletal system organizes itself to move a body through space.

Just as high school science courses will prepare you for the rigorous science requirements of a physical therapy degree program, writing, literature, psychology, and history courses will expand your understanding of people and your ability to communicate and connect with others. Physical therapy requires both a scientific and a human approach.

Getting the Right Education and Training

To become a PT or a PTA, you must meet very specific educational requirements, which are laid down by the APTA. Remember, even though PTs and PTAs work together, the responsibilities and the education required for the two jobs are very different. PTs must earn a master's degree from a college or university. PTAs must earn an associate's degree from a community or junior college.

Earning a Degree as a Physical Therapist

To become a PT, students must earn a master's degree from an accredited collegiate physical therapy program. Recently, some schools have started to offer an entry-level doctorate degree instead of the master's. This may become more common in the future. An "entry-level" degree means the beginning degree in the profession that allows you to qualify to take the national exam and to become a licensed, practicing physical therapist.

There are also advanced academic degrees that concentrate on certain specialties or qualify you to do specialized research or become a professor. These advanced degrees are beyond the scope of this book, however. The information given here is concerned with getting you going in the field; later, it will be up to you to determine whether you want to commit yourself to further formal study. For more information, contact the APTA or a university with a physical therapy department.

One thing is certain: Even if you never pursue an advanced degree, as a PT you are committing yourself to lifelong learning. You will learn on the job, and you probably will take many continuing education courses. The entry-level master's or doctorate degree is the beginning; it's a way into the profession. Once you're in, you will have many avenues of education and growth from which to choose.

Some programs that offer the entry-level master's degree are six- or seven-year programs that you can enter right after high school. Others are two-year programs designed for students who have already earned a college degree and are ready for the professional phase of physical therapy training. Ask your high school or college career counselor or other job counselor to help you sort out all the options and find out about fees, financial aid, and scholarship programs. You can find a listing of accredited physical therapy degree programs at the APTA Web site.

Entry-Level Master's Degree

In a physical therapy program at a college or university that offers the entry-level master's degree and accepts students right out of high school, students pursue a major of their choice for the first three years. They also must fulfill tough prerequisites in the sciences. Some students may choose to major in athletic training and eventually become both a certified athletic trainer and a licensed PT. In the fourth year, they start taking the physical therapy courses that will prepare them for the profession.

In deciding who will be admitted to the program, many factors are considered: grades from high school, particularly in science courses; SAT or ACT scores; letters of recommendation; an evaluation of a student's commitment and high-school extracurricular activities; and an essay stating why the student wants to become a PT. If you are accepted into the six-year program, during your first years in college you will be expected to observe or volunteer in a physical therapy department. You must keep up your grades if you want to continue on the physical therapy track and eventually start the professional phase of the program.

Getting a Bachelor's Degree First · me. thats me.

You also may wait until you are ready to graduate from college to apply to a physical therapy program. Once you have earned a four-year college degree and have taken the required college science courses, you may apply to a program that lasts two or three years and starts you right off in the professional phase of the training.

Schools that accept people who have already earned a college degree accept an applicant based on an evaluation of the applicant's college record, an essay about why the applicant wants to become a PT, an interview, letters of recommendation, and the completion of a certain number of hours of observation, volunteer work, or paid work as an aide. Some programs require these hours to have been spent in at least two different physical therapy settings. The bachelor's degree of an applicant may be in any major—biology and psychology are popular choices. Students in the two- or three-year programs are of varying ages.

Every program is different. What follows is one way a university might schedule its coursework during the professional phase.

1. The first semester is theoretically and scientifically based. Students take courses in human anatomy, neuroscience, and kinesiology. They take a practice-oriented class in examination and evaluation and also study physical therapy procedures, including how to get patients walking, massage, and transfers (helping patients get from a bed to a wheelchair, for instance). They also take a seminar on how to conduct physical therapy research.

2. During the second semester, students learn how to apply physical therapy modalities, and they take two survey courses, one in pathology, or disease, and the other in orthopedic and neurological disorders. They also study cardiopulmonary physiology.

3. The third semester is very treatment-oriented. Subjects covered are orthopedic and neurological physical therapy. Courses in pediatric physical therapy and prosthetics and orthotics are also required.

4. More coursework on orthopedics is completed in the fourth semester. Other classes include physical therapy management, geriatrics, and psychology.

5. Some schools require that students complete a research thesis. This involves setting up an experiment or research study, using either their fellow classmates or a patient population as subjects.

Alex

Alex Bagley already had a college degree when he decided to become a PT, but he had not completed all the science courses that he needed to get into a two-year physical therapy degree program. He had to complete courses in math, physics, chemistry, and biology while he continued to work at his job at *Time* magazine. It wasn't easy. He was turned down by a couple of schools, but Alex was accepted by the physical therapy program at the State University of New York at Stony Brook. Getting to Stony Brook involved a six-hour-a-day commute and getting up at 4 AM. But the two years went by quickly, according to Alex, and the schooling he got was rigorous and top-notch. One of his first courses was anatomy, which included dissection.

> You are issued a human cadaver—a brand-new, untouched cadaver. I happened to be in the lab late at night, sipping a cup of coffee and dissecting my cadaver's wrist extensors, and I looked around and thought, "Wow, I'm the only thing that's alive here and I'm in a room with twenty-five corpses." But I liked it so much that it didn't bother me. We hold someone's brain. The technician will cut off the top of the skull and remove

the brain and here it is for you to dissect, and you know that somebody's life, somebody's soul, somebody's personality was in this. This tissue was what held it. It's very strange in a way, but it's fascinating.

Clinical Affiliations—a Chance to Practice

Throughout PT and PTA school, courses include both academic classes and labs, in which students turn theory into practice. Usually they work on each other: One plays the role of patient, and one assumes the duties of the PT.

There are also full-time clinical affiliations. These are eight-week opportunities to do the job for real, and they are tremendously valuable learning experiences for the physical therapy student.

The timing differs from school to school, but students often participate in their first practicum, or clinical affiliation program, during the summer before the final year of the program. The second half of the final year is devoted to two more eight-week affiliations. Sometimes, students travel to different parts of the country to work, observe, and train in hospitals, rehabilitation centers, and outpatient clinics. Other times, they stay in the area, especially if the college is in a big city with many major health care settings nearby.

During these clinical affiliations, students are supervised by, work alongside, and learn from the PTs who are employed in the various health care settings. PTs teach students the art and science of physical therapy and pass along the knowledge from one generation to another, with the experienced PTs serving as teachers, role models, and mentors to the students.

Tracy

Tracy Sawyer traveled to New York City, Baltimore, and Pittsfield, Massachusetts, for her affiliations. Students have to find and pay for their own housing, she says, although the affiliation site may have a list of apartments that are available. Sometimes there are residences connected to the site, where physical therapy students can live.

Tracy says that the quality of an affiliation experience can vary according to the attitude of the physical therapy clinical instructor to whom the student is assigned. Tracy remembers that on one of her affiliations, she had a couple of instructors who weren't very helpful.

> Every day I would go in and they would quiz me on things. They were not being instructors so much as drill sergeants. A good instructor works with the student but also lets the student learn to do things on his or her own. On the other hand, sometimes instructors give you free rein. Well, students don't really know anything, so that's definitely not a good idea! The best is when you're with someone who you know really likes what he or she does—he or she has a lot of knowledge, is confident in what he or she does, and teaches you but doesn't just spoon-feed you.

Chris

Chris Barrett did her first affiliation at a big-city hospital. Her second affiliation was at a small, Catholic hospital in New Jersey where some of the PTs knew the patients because they all came from the same neighborhood.

It was interesting to see the difference between a big, impersonal teaching hospital where people came expecting the doctors to be at the top of their game, and a community hospital, serving an elderly Italian and younger Hispanic community, where there weren't the fancy doctors, but where they had much better nursing care. I never saw a person with a bed-sore at St. Mary's.

I learned a lot about patient care. If you're not sensitive, you're not going to get any-where. Your skills are meaningless if you don't know who your patient is and what your patient wants.

Getting Licensed as a Physical Therapist

After students complete their coursework and clinical affiliations and graduate from a physical therapy program, they must take the national examination in physical therapy to become licensed PTs in their states. The exam is a written test that lasts for a full day. For information about the exam, contact the APTA.

Studying to Be a PTA

Physical therapist assistant programs take two years to complete and are usually offered at community colleges or at schools of health sciences. Graduates receive an associate's degree as a PTA. The programs require a mixture of liberal arts and science courses. There are also many clinical classes and labs.

You can enter these programs straight out of high school or later in life. The APTA lists schools that offer the PTA degree on its Web site.

Every PTA program is a little different. Be sure to have someone at each school to which you apply go over that school's requirements, certification status, and curriculum with you. Check the certification status of the school. Perhaps your high school guidance counselor can help you navigate the process of applying to schools and inquiring about costs, scholarships, and financial aid.

PTA students receive their education through course work and their clinical fieldwork training under the supervision of experienced PTAs and PTs.

Margaret Plack, who is head of both the PT and PTA programs at Touro College in New York City, cautions that, "Some people think that an associate's degree program should be easy, but it is an intensive program; they're here full days, and it's a lot of work."

Of course, every school has its own admissions policy, but at most schools, applicants are required to submit a high school diploma or a GED, an essay about why they want to become a PTA, documentation of a specified number of hours of volunteer experience, and two letters of recommendation. Some applicants may have to take a placement exam. Applicants also will be interviewed and evaluated for pertinent life experience.

Once admitted to the program, students will take classes that cover academics such as biology, anatomy, physiology, psychology, kinesiology, and writing. Clinically oriented classes cover topics such as cardiopulmonary pathology and treatment, the aging process,

musculoskeletal and neurological problems and rehabilitation, training in the use of modalities, and ethics.
Students also complete clinical internships in a variety
of health care settings, including hospitals, nursing
homes, clinics, and rehabilitation centers.

PTA Certification

In some states, PTAs must take an exam and be
licensed. In others, no exam is required, but you must
apply for certification after graduating from an
accredited PTA school. Contact the APTA or call your
state's licensure board to find out what the rules are
where you live.

Everyone Is Encouraged to Apply

The field of physical therapy is wide open for recruit-
ing more people from minority backgrounds. More
PTs and PTAs who speak Spanish or who are bilingual
are needed. Statistics show that by 2025, at least half of
the children born in the United States will be of
minority backgrounds. This shows the need to incorporate more students from minority backgrounds into
medical professions. PTs want to reach people in all
neighborhoods, and they want a profession that repre-
sents all Americans.

Marquette University, in Milwaukee, Wisconsin, is one
college that has instituted programs to recruit and give
academic and financial opportunities to young people
from minority and/or disadvantaged backgrounds.

Marquette offers seven-week mentoring programs for local high school kids, teaming each one with a physical therapy student. The university also has a summer science program for college students who are interested in transferring into the Marquette physical therapy program, and it offers academic and financial support to minority and disadvantaged physical therapy students.

The APTA has a mentoring program, called Early Professional Socialization Experience, or EPSE. EPSE connects minority students interested in physical therapy to a mentor, or adviser, who assists them with admission into a physical therapy program. The program provides career support and guidance for those who are identified as promising students and future PTs.

Working in
a Hospital

By the time you graduate from a PT or PTA program, you will have received an all-around physical therapy education and worked in a variety of different health care settings during your full-time clinical affiliations or internships. When you receive your degree, if you're a PT you will take the national exam and apply for a license to practice in your state. If you have been trained as a PTA, you will follow the procedures for practicing as a PTA in your state.

Once you are legally able to practice, you will start making your own way within the profession. That's usually not too difficult to do. You will have connections from your affiliations and internships, and, as Margaret Plack puts it, "The world of physical therapy is small, and people know people that know people." While the world of physical therapy may be small, as a field it is wide; there are many different types of opportunities and many different paths you can follow.

One of the first choices will be where you want to work. Hospital? Clinic? Nursing home? School? Private office? Rehabilitation hospital? Later, after you've worked in one type of setting for a while, you may want to try a different sort of place; at some point, you may even be in a position to start up your own practice as a PT. One PT interviewed for this book says she has had a "checkered" career. Usually that's considered a bad thing—"checkered" means that you've hopped around the board like a checker, done a little of this and a little of that, and it hasn't really amounted to much. But in physical therapy, many PTs and PTAs have done different kinds of satisfying work in various places, and so "checkered" might mean that your career has a lot of variety, color, and breadth.

One setting in which practice covers all of these areas is a hospital. Practically everyone works in a hospital during one of their clinical affiliations while they are in PT school, and for many a job at a hospital is their first job in physical therapy. Some PTs and PTAs practice at hospitals for the whole of their careers.

Only at a hospital can you see such a variety of patients and problems under one roof. Hospital doctors—physiatrists, who specialize in rehabilitation, as well as cardiologists, orthopedic physicians, and others—issue orders for physical therapy for their patients.

PTs who work in hospitals have rotations, which means that they rotate through several specialty areas. Chris Barrett knew that she eventually wanted to work with dancers in a performing-arts practice, but early on she worked in a big-city hospital and says the experience was very important.

"I liked being around doctors and having a dialogue with other health professionals, and understanding where I fit into the structure of American medicine," she says. "I thought it was important to be comfortable in a hospital with all the white coats, even in an operating room, and to recognize what a really sick person looks like and be comfortable around disability. I think that has definitely helped me in my career because even though now I usually treat people who are basically healthy, you still want to be able to deal with people along the whole spectrum of health."

The major goal of a physical therapist who works at a hospital is to get his or her patients well and independent enough to return home or be transferred to another live-in setting. Following are just some of the jobs that a PT, assisted by a PTA, might do in a large hospital.

Bedside

Before and after operations, and when people need to move their bodies but are too weak to go to the physical therapy gym, treatment is given in the patients' rooms. The first steps may be to work on sitting up in bed or transferring to a chair. Walking, or gait training, is central to regaining independence.

Neurological

The neurological rotation is often part of bedside. In neurological, PTs work with people who have traumatic brain injuries, strokes, and spinal cord injuries. Stroke patients may suffer paralysis and lose contact with parts of their bodies because of a sudden blockage of blood and oxygen to the brain. For instance, they may not be aware that they have a left arm or a left leg because all the information routes that go from the brain to that side have been damaged.

In those cases, a PT needs to make the patient aware that he or she has limbs. The PT would encourage the patient to put weight on the leg or arm to get sensation going. The neurological part of physical therapy is a mystery of sorts; evaluating and treating the patient is kind of like putting together a puzzle.

Orthopedic

Patients on this rotation may have had hip, knee, or shoulder replacements, or surgeries to fix badly fractured bones. The goal is to get them started on physical therapy, which is mostly aimed at strengthening the muscles that surround the area that was operated on. People with orthopedic problems make up a large percentage of the people who are treated by PTs in all settings. After their operations—often in as little time as two or three days—orthopedic patients will be sent home or to a rehab facility to receive many more weeks of physical therapy. Orthopedics is further explained in chapter 11.

Cardiopulmonary

Patients who have undergone heart bypass or heart valve replacement surgery need physical therapy to recover. They need to be started on a carefully supervised, graduated program of activity and exercise. Sometimes they may need what is called pulmonary toileting to get the secretions out of their lungs. PTs help people to cough, teach them how to position themselves so their lungs don't fill with fluid, and may perform percussion and vibration (tapping parts of the body) to loosen fluids in their chests.

Trauma Center

Some hospitals have trauma centers where people who have been seriously injured—often in car accidents—

are cared for once their condition is stabilized. These patients are in critical condition, often with multiple injuries. Tracy Sawyer worked for a while at a trauma center. Part of what Tracy did was respiratory work, like percussion and vibration to clear the lungs. Tracy says even those in a coma needed their limbs taken through a range of motion. If the patients had brain or spinal cord injuries, their limbs might have been pulled up and bent, and could get stuck that way, so Tracy would help the nurse to position them better. Patients who are conscious are started on breathing and muscle exercises, and are helped to start sitting up in bed.

Burns

Burn wounds must be treated quickly because, even though it takes the skin and the tissues a long time to heal, things start to tighten up quickly. Burn victims often have skin grafted (transplanted) onto the damaged area by a physician. Once a graft has been put on a part of the body, that part has to be immobilized for five days so it can be accepted by the body.

PTs get burn patients moving or splinted in some way so that if they can't move, at least their skin won't tighten up. Splints are made from thermoplastics. When put in hot water, the plastic becomes soft and the PT can custom-make the splint for the patient. PTs also can make airplane splints to keep a person's shoulders and trunk from moving.

Amputations

Sometimes a person loses a limb in an accident, but more often the cause is severe diabetes or extreme circulatory problems. If a person's leg can't get enough blood and oxygen, sores appear, the tissues become infected or die, and a surgeon may have to amputate the leg.

For six months, Chris Barrett worked in a hospital's amputee clinic, helping people learn to walk on their artificial legs, or prostheses:

> The insurance people won't send patients to inpatient rehab if they don't feel they have a shot at healing well. If the amputation is below the knee, they can almost always learn to walk. I had a reputation for never giving up on anybody. It's a big energy demand, to stand on a prosthesis, so I ended up doing a lot of cardiac stuff, too. Amputees have to build up their hearts, and they can't do it on a bicycle, so they use an upper body ergometer, which is like an arm bicycle.

Intensive Care Unit

PTs may work in the intensive care unit (ICU), helping to position the patients or gently moving their arms and legs. These PTs must be able to work surrounded by tubes and wires, and they must know a lot about the machinery and the meaning of all the information that is constantly being generated about the patients' conditions.

Other Places PTs and PTAs Practice

10

PTs and PTAs work in many different kinds of places. We've already seen examples of patients who receive physical therapy while they are in the hospital so they can regain enough strength, stamina, and physical independence to be discharged and return home.

But if a young working woman is in pain—feeling a twinge in her hip after a snowboarding accident, for example—a short course of treatment with a PT who works in a sports therapy clinic right down the road may be all that is needed.

For other people, physical problems may be present from birth, or soon after. For instance, if young children with cerebral palsy are not able to reach out, touch, and interact with their toys, that inability may create a gap not only in physical development, but in the development of curiosity, thinking, and enthusiasm as well. These kids will benefit if they are enrolled in a special school, where they can work with a PT and receive the attention of a whole team of therapists, doctors, and teachers.

For competitive athletes, a PT may be a trusted adviser, and some PTs are right at the front lines at the Olympic and the Goodwill Games, treating and helping to train the participating athletes.

Clinics

Some clinics are affiliated with hospitals; others are privately owned. Many PTs and PTAs work in clinics and help people with a wide range of health problems. These people are living at home and come into the clinic for physical therapy treatments.

Rehabilitation Hospitals and Centers

Many PTs, PTAs, and aides work at rehabilitation facilities. Regular hospitals offer mostly acute, short-term care, but most patients who are treated in rehabilitation hospitals or centers need a longer period of more concentrated care. Rehabilitation hospitals, as we discussed in chapter 3, use a team approach, and they treat problems such as strokes, chronic pain, brain injury, severe orthopedic injury, spinal cord injury, and cardiac rehabilitation.

Tracy Sawyer worked for twelve years as part of a team at a rehabilitation hospital. She worked with many different types of patients and was exposed to a lot of different things. Some of her patients had suffered spinal cord injuries in automobile accidents or other catastrophic events. Tracy had wanted to help people with spinal cord injuries ever since she first decided to become a PT, and she was doing it. At the same time, she took many continuing education courses in spinal injury care.

Some of Tracy's patients who had spinal cord injuries no longer had normal sensation, and sometimes they felt as though their feet were on fire. Tracy worked to relieve their pain, often using different modalities. Teaching people ways to stay mobile was all-important.

PTs teach people the basics of mobility, whether that involves teaching them how to get out of bed, how to move around in bed, how to get in and out of a wheelchair, how to get on and off the toilet, how to use a wheelchair, or how to hold their balance getting in and out of a car. It might mean teaching someone else to make them mobile. A PT might work with someone who is so paralyzed that he or she is on a respirator, teaching the patient's caregivers how to assist him or her. Patients who are on a respirator can be taught to propel a wheelchair using a special device controlled by their mouths or their heads. Of course, some patients have incomplete injuries and can learn to walk again.

Tracy says there's always a reward to rehabilitation because you're always seeing something new happen, even if it's the littlest thing.

Other Rehabilitation Team Members

If you are interested in working in a rehabilitation hospital or center, you might want to learn more about the other professionals who work on such teams. Rehabilitation team members include:

Physiatrists

A physiatrist is a medical doctor who is a specialist in rehabilitation and physical medicine. Physiatrists work in hospitals, rehabilitation centers, and private offices. Often, they are the rehabilitation team's leader. They manage and coordinate the treatment of people with acute and chronic pain and serious disability. Their methods and philosophy are very similar to those of PTs in that they emphasize working to improve their patients' function and quality of life through nonsurgical means. Physiatrists often work closely with PTs and often refer their patients to PTs for treatment. Because physiatrists are MDs, they can do certain things that PTs can't, like prescribe pain medications and perform certain kinds of tests. For more information about physiatrists and the medical specialty of physical medicine and rehabilitation, contact the American Academy of Physical Medicine and Rehabilitation at (312) 464-9700, or log on to their Web site at www.aapmr.org.

Other Medical Doctors

Besides physiatrists, other types of doctors may be members or leaders of the rehabilitation team. These doctors may be primary care physicians, neurologists (doctors who specialize in brain and nervous system disorders and injuries), pediatricians (doctors who treat children), orthopedists (doctors who specialize in muscles and bones), or other specialists. To find out more about becoming a medical doctor, contact the American Medical Association through its Web site, www.ama-assn.org.

Occupational Therapists

These therapists, known as OTs, often work closely with PTs, although occupational therapy has a different focus. In addition to working to improve a patient's physical well-being, OTs address psychological, social, and environmental factors in their treatments. They often help patients with the fine movements of the hands and arms, and may offer special assistance in learning skills that lead to productive, independent, and satisfying lives. OTs also have expertise in helping people engage in social and creative activities, and they devise and make special equipment that patients may need to perform activities of daily living. They usually have a solid background in psychology. OTs now graduate with a bachelor's degree in occupational therapy, but by 2007, an entry-level master's degree will be required. OTs must pass a national examination to become certified. Occupational therapy assistants must earn an associate's degree in occupational therapy. For more information, contact the American Occupational Therapy Association through its Web site, www.aota.org, or by calling (301) 652-2682.

Orthotists and Prosthetists

Orthotists fit, design, and construct braces. Prosthetists fit, design, and construct artificial limbs for people with amputations. For instance, a person who has had a leg amputated because of diabetes or poor circulation can be fitted with a temporary prosthesis. Then the PT will help the person learn to walk with the artificial leg. The prosthetist will then make a permanent prosthesis, which will look much like a real leg. The prosthetist also follows up and consults with the PT to make sure the fit is right, and makes modifications in the prosthesis to make it more comfortable and efficient for the wearer.

Other Rehabilitation Team Members

Other members of the rehabilitation team include social workers, psychologists, rehabilitation nurses, speech therapists, and recreational therapists.

Schools

Many private and state-owned schools exist for children who have physical and developmental problems. Often, these schools employ PTs to work with the students both in groups and one-on-one. Pedriatric physical therapy is discussed in more detail in chapter 12.

Nursing Homes

Many PTs work for nursing homes, helping elderly residents recovering from accidents or surgery, and also just working to keep them mobile. Working in geriatrics is further discussed in chapter 12.

Treating People in Their Homes

Although most people receive physical therapy in hospitals, rehab facilities, nursing homes, clinics, and privately owned offices, some PTs bring their skills to patients at their homes.

Home health agencies hire PTs to visit people who have difficulty getting to a clinic or private office on a regular basis, or who are homebound. Many of these patients are elderly, and most of them have recently returned home from the hospital. There are also home health programs for very young children who need physical therapy.

One advantage to treating someone in his or her home is that the PT can actually see how the home is set up and what tasks the patient needs to accomplish. PTs can help people regain and retain their mobility, and teach people ways to conserve energy and avoid falls. Just doing simple ROM exercises or gentle strengthening can raise a person's spirits, as well as improve his or her functioning.

Some PTs are directly employed by home health agencies; others may work through an agency as independent contractors, and still others may be hired privately, meaning the patient pays out of his or her pocket. When Tracy Sawyer started her family, she wanted to work part-time. Now she works three days a week as an independent contractor through a home health agency, and she can usually make her own hours.

Owning Your Own Business

Some physical therapists own their own businesses, and for many younger PTs, it is a cherished goal for the future. Establishing a private practice takes courage, good connections, and start-up money, but it allows a PT to focus the practice to reflect his or her special interests and abilities. If the venture proves successful, the PT will reap the rewards—professional, personal, and financial.

Tim

Tim Tyler recently opened his own sports therapy office in Westchester County, New York. He formed a private corporation, or PC. Tim bought a computer program on how to develop a business plan, and he read a lot of small business, accounting, and marketing books. He focused on his budget: where the money would come from and where it would go. After scouting the area for a space, Tim found one he liked and rented it. He plans to keep his overhead low, and his wife—who is his receptionist—will be his only employee. Tim has contacts with doctors in the area who will send him patients. Opening a business isn't hard, Tim says. What is hard is staying open! But he's confident that he will make it work and says it's important for future PTs to realize that the opportunity is out there to own a private practice.

Orthopedic Physical Therapy and Its Offshoots

11

The physical therapy specialty with the largest number of PTs is orthopedics, a branch of medicine that deals with muscles, bones, tendons, joints, and ligaments. These are the parts of our anatomy that allow us to move, stand, bend, walk, jump, skip, squat, gallop, lie down, climb, reach, and sit at a desk—they make up the musculoskeletal system. Musculoskeletal problems include arthritis, lower back pain, and injuries like bone fractures, sprains, tendonitis, strains, and torn ligaments.

Orthopedic physical therapy is practiced in all physical therapy workplaces, but it dominates the scene at most outpatient facilities, sports medicine clinics, and private offices because people who have orthopedic injuries or chronic orthopedic problems are often well enough to live at home.

Orthopedic Injuries

Injuries can be divided into two categories: traumatic and those caused by overuse or incorrect movement. A car accident is a traumatic event and may cause traumatic orthopedic injuries like broken bones or whiplash. Sometimes traumatic injuries occur because of accidents at work. Injuries that are due to overuse or misuse may be the final result of a long-term pattern of incorrect movement habits. These overuse or misuse injuries can happen on the job, while doing housework or deskwork, or while playing sports or musical instruments. These are the kinds of injuries that are, ideally, preventable. PTs can treat both types of injuries. They also can teach people new movement skills and instruct them how to perform their activities more safely.

Arthritis

About one in six people in the United States is affected by arthritis. Arthritis is the medical term for more than 100 diseases and disorders that cause joints to become damaged or inflamed, resulting in pain and stiffness. In the most common form, called osteoarthritis, bones and cartilage deteriorate, partly as a result of the aging process, and the result is pain and stiffness. So far, there is no cure for arthritis, but PTs use modalities, mobilization, and exercise to decrease pain, increase ROM of the joints, and increase strength. PTs also teach patients how they can decrease the pressure on their joints as they move and perform everyday activities. Physicians who specialize in treating arthritis are known as rheumatologists, but if a person with arthritis needs an operation—a hip replacement, for instance—an orthopedic surgeon will perform the procedure.

Presurgery and Postsurgery

Orthopedic PTs often work in cooperation with orthopedic surgeons. Often, a surgeon will refer a patient to a PT to see if the injury or condition will respond to physical therapy alone. When orthopedic operations are necessary, patients are sent to physical therapy afterward to strengthen the surrounding muscles and regain mobility.

There are many different orthopedic surgeries, including "cleaning out" joints, resetting broken bones, mending fractures with metal screws, and replacing shoulder, knee, and hip joints with devices made of plastic and steel. Surgery isn't an easy fix; working with a PT for some weeks or months is essential to recovery. Many patients have their first taste of physical therapy at the hospital, but soon some of them may be home and starting physical therapy at an outpatient facility. Others will go to live at a rehabilitation hospital for a time, where they can be cared for and do physical therapy until they are capable of living independently.

Lower Back Pain

Lower back pain is the most common cause of disability in people under the age of forty-five. According to the National Institute of Neurological Disorders and Stroke, it is a symptom that can arise from many causes. It can range from a dull ache to absolute agony. In the past, the main treatment was bed rest, but now medical professionals recognize that mobilization, back stabilization and conditioning exercises, and patient education are the best remedies. There is no one more qualified than a PT to apply these three remedies, and PTs and PTAs treat a lot of patients who suffer from back pain.

Ergonomics

Some rehabilitation centers or on-site clinics in industrial and corporate workplaces offer a range of services to help people return to work after an injury. At a rehabilitation center in Chicago, PTs work as part of a team to evaluate a patient's strength, flexibility, and ability to perform the tasks associated with his or her job. Once the team has identified a patient's assets and deficits, PTs create an individualized program to improve the skills needed to return to work. Treatment programs combine exercises and education to help people improve their physical functioning, as well as decrease any strain or stress that their everyday tasks place upon them.

Conditions treated include carpal tunnel syndrome, tendonitis, and chronic pain in the neck and trunk. Treatment may include ergonomic education, which teaches people how to adjust the equipment they use on the job so they can work more safely and comfortably. Sometimes a company will hire a clinic or health care company to manage industrial testing and rehabilitation programs for its employees.

Orthopedics is what most people think of when they hear the words "physical therapy." Across all the different places where physical therapy is practiced, orthopedic problems make up a large portion of problems that PTs and PTAs treat. But other specialties have emerged from within orthopedic physical therapy, such as sports therapy, hand therapy, manual therapy, and performing-arts therapy.

Sports Therapy

Orthopedic PTs who specialize in treating the injuries of active people and athletes call themselves sports therapists. Sports therapy spans the fields of physical therapy and sports medicine.

Sports therapists have physical therapy skills plus special expertise in sports and sports injuries. They work with professional and amateur athletes, and treat other active individuals as well. PTs who specialize in sports medicine often practice at privately owned or hospital-connected sports medicine clinics, or sometimes at fitness facilities and health clubs.

The thing that sets sports therapy apart is that the patients are generally active and body-oriented; they may be able to rehabilitate much faster and more completely than those who may have other health problems or are used to a more sedentary lifestyle.

A sports PT first works with the athlete to prevent injury; then if the athlete does get hurt, the sports PT evaluates the injury, treats it, and rehabilitates it. When the rehabilitation is complete, it's back to prevention. Active people don't want to stop doing their sports or their workouts. They continue to educate themselves about how to avoid injury. A sports PT can help balance the patient's love of sports and need for healthy exercise with a sensible, physically aware approach that will minimize injury and overuse.

In sports therapy, it is very important to figure out why a certain injury happened, or why a certain joint is chronically painful, because a PT wants to make sure that it doesn't recur. A PT aims to change the way the person is playing the sport or doing the aerobics class so that he or she can avoid injuries.

"Most critical to preventing injury and getting the most out of your swimming routine is concentrating on your stroke," says Sheila Klausner, the Sydney 2000 U.S. Olympic swim team's official PT. "Good stroke technique is critical. If you maintain good form, you will reduce your risk of injuring joints and muscles." The swim team's daily training regimen consisted of two sets of practice sessions and three physical therapy sessions. Sheila says:

> Without adequate care while competing, Olympic swimmers can run the risk that a small injury, or even simple physical fatigue, will affect their performances. Much of what I do consists of stretching exercises for the ligaments and tendons, and therapeutic massage to keep the muscles loose and ready for heavy exertion.

Tim

Tim Tyler majored in athletic training in college. Athletic trainers have many physical therapy skills, and they are on the scene when an athlete is first injured; many certified athletic trainers, or ATCs, work for high schools and college athletic departments. Tim covered swimming, baseball, and football, and did a lot of taping and bracing to prevent injury, as well as providing immediate, on-the-spot treatment for injuries.

One of the clinical affiliations he did to earn his athletic training certificate was at a physical therapy clinic. At the clinic, the PTs were treating not just team athletes but all sorts of patients with sports-related injuries—amateur athletes, so-called weekend warriors, who had pushed themselves too hard, and sixty-five-year-old people who had shoulder pain because they were swinging the golf club incorrectly. Tim was hooked.

> I said to myself, "Wow—this is the role of the physical therapist—it's more than waiting around for something that might go wrong at a game or a practice, it's more proactive." I saw what PTs were doing with all ages and all populations, and the intimacy the therapist has with his patients when he treats them with hands-on manual therapy—you don't get that so much as an ATC.

Tim wound up becoming an ATC and then going on to a two-year, entry-level master's program in physical therapy. For his PT school research thesis, he did a study of back pain in ice hockey players, testing the flexibility of their hips and trying to relate that to which of the players suffered from back pain. He happened to connect with someone at Nicholas Institute of Sports Medicine and Athletic Trauma (NISMAT) who was associated with the New York Rangers ice hockey team, and was invited to get his sample of players from that team. When the directors at NISMAT saw how interested Tim was in physical therapy and how much he loved his work, they hired him; he started to practice sports physical therapy and conduct sports medicine research at NISMAT.

One important thing about sports therapy is an increased emphasis on patient responsibility. Tim Tyler says: "We don't do a lot of 'TLC' (tender loving care); we do a lot of 'You're responsible for getting yourself better.' I'm a teacher more than anything. I teach you how to help yourself."

Manual Therapy

Every PT uses some manual therapy. Formal manual therapy is a way of treating patients that has been refined and expanded by some PTs who treat delicate orthopedic problems. To become a really good manual therapist takes special training, years of experience, and—if you're lucky—a work situation where you can have an on-the-job apprenticeship. Chris Barrett says:

> It takes a long time to learn to feel this stuff; when you're out there by yourself, you can be feeling around in [the tissues of] someone's ankle and think, "Is that because the joint is blocked? Is that a tight muscle or a loose ligament?"
>
> The people I work with are a resource for me because they're so experienced and so skilled . . . I feel like the rest of the world is speeding up, but one of the things I love about my job is that the more I slow down, the better I do. This kind of work makes you really slow down and focus, and I like that.

Performing-Arts Therapy

Whether practicing or performing, dancers and musicians run the risk of overuse and strain. There is also, at times, a psychological strain associated with performance, and stage fright or anxiety can make the body tense up and result in injury or fatigue.

Performing-arts physical therapists work in private offices and also work under contract to organizations like ballet companies and music schools. Chris Barrett works with the dancers of the New York City Ballet and the students at the Juilliard School of Music. She says ballet, for example, can take a tremendous toll on the body. The female dancers are working up on their toes and with extreme ranges of motion. The male dancers lift the women and execute great leaps and jumps. A professional ballet dancer works six days a week, and the typical workday includes an hour-long class in the morning, a rehearsal from 1:00 to 7:00 PM, and an evening performance.

Chris and the other PTs she works with are able to prevent injury in the dancers by treating problems promptly and correcting habits that lead to misuse and overuse of the muscles, ligaments, and tendons. Chris says, "I think the whole point of ballet technique used to be transcending your body. The romantic ideal was this weightless, boneless sylph, flitting across the stage and having no gravity. I think over the last twenty years, people are realizing that if they recognize their musculoskeletal limits, they can dance longer and have happier, healthier careers."

Musicians may be at risk for cumulative trauma disorders, or CTDs, which are caused by factors such as repetition, fatigue, force, and static or awkward posture. Common CTDs include tendonitis, carpal tunnel syndrome, fibromyalgia, and bursitis. Even transporting an instrument from place to place can be a physical demand on the musician and can cause injury. A PT can treat and prevent such disorders and strains.

Other Specialties

12

Although orthopedics is perhaps the largest branch of physical therapy, there are other groups that require a PT with special training. Children, the elderly, and women, for instance, all have challenges unique to them. PTs can obtain further education or training to become specialists in these areas.

Working with Children—Pediatrics

PTs and PTAs work with infants and children who have disabilities from birth or who are seriously ill or injured. They work in children's hospitals, regular or special schools, or in private practices. They also work with kids—abled and disabled—who play sports. Some PTs who work with children are members of the APTA's pediatric section.

Margaret

Margaret Plack always knew she wanted to work with children. Her first PT job was at a cerebral palsy day center and school, where she worked with children and adults who had cerebral palsy, brain injuries, or other neurological problems. The children's section was a school for kids from only a few months old to age twenty-one. U.S. law states that every child is entitled to an appropriate education, whether it's a child who is developing typically or a child who needs special services in a school for kids with disabilities. Some of the kids Margaret worked with were mentally retarded; others, she says, were "as bright as could be." They had problems coordinating their muscles, and many were unable to walk. With cerebral palsy, the muscles contract, and physical therapy can help to release these contractures and prevent them from worsening. The goal at the school was to help each child reach his or her maximum potential. This might be by helping a child to walk, to graduate from the school, or to move into a mainstream school.

Margaret worked as a member of a team that included physicians, teachers, nurses, occupational therapists, speech therapists, and others. She also worked with people who make orthotics because many of the children needed special supports in their shoes to position the foot and prevent deformities.

Margaret worked with kids right in the classroom and was always in close communication with the parents. Sometimes she would work one-on-one with a child in the gym. The gym was full of big balls and toys.

Kids would lie over a large, plastic physioball on their bellies or backs, moving and stretching with Margaret's hands-on help.

> My job was to make things easier for them, and I never believed in letting them cry. If they cried from frustration, something was too hard for them and I had to change my approach. Some of the sessions were spent just comforting the children, to help them go on.

The whole rehabilitation team was assigned to a classroom, and they all would sit down once a week, discussing any problems and making improvements in the way the classroom was being run.

One of the reasons Margaret became a PT instead of a physician was that she wanted to develop more of a long-term relationship with her patients, and working with children, she certainly has that.

> There are some children I've seen over thirteen or fourteen years, and I've seen them really develop. They've become part of my family, and I've become part of their families, that's how close some of the relationships become. Suppose my new patient is a two-and-a-half-year-old child, who is very attached to his mom and is used to doctors poking and prodding. And here I'm supposed to work with this child who doesn't want to get out of Mom's lap because he just got out of the hospital. Part of the art of being a physical therapist is being

able to establish that relationship, and key to that relationship is the development of trust.

So, with that youngster I have to develop some degree of trust before he is willing to come and work with me. With any age kid, I can have a goal. I can decide that I want to work on walking today, but if the child comes in and doesn't want to stand, but does want to sit at the bench and do something else, well then, I have to do that because I have to respect that child.

Later in her career, Margaret became supervisor at the same school and day center. She coordinated schedules and classes, met with parents, worked on funding, and taught the younger PTs and PT students.

Working with the Elderly—Geriatrics

Physical therapists work with older adults in a variety of settings. For instance, sports therapists are seeing more sports injuries in people over the age of sixty-five; in one way, that's a promising trend because it means that more older people are keeping active. Older people also see PTs in private clinics and outpatient facilities, and many are treated at home (through home health agencies) or cared for in nursing homes. Aging brings with it many challenges. Each individual is different, but older people can benefit from physical therapy, whether they are active or frail. Physical therapy may prevent lifelong disability and restore the highest level of functioning.

Older people can be affected by a number of specific diseases and conditions that can be treated and improved with physical therapy. These conditions and diseases include osteoporosis, Parkinson's disease, hip fractures, and incontinence. We've already seen how physical therapists can help treat arthritis and strokes.

No physical therapists are more devoted to prevention strategies than those who work with older adults. They can see that if a person has been inactive for his whole life, he will have a much harder time as he ages and may develop multiple health problems. No one can totally escape the limits of age or the reality that life comes to an end, but proper physical care and activity can prove to be a comfort and a help.

In nursing homes, PTs and PTAs work to keep even the frailest of their patients mobile. If patients must lie in bed for long periods of time, or if they are too weak to shift their positions, they can develop bed sores. Many PTs have special skills in wound healing. PTs and PTAs also teach people how to transfer from their beds to a chair or wheelchair. Even in those over the age of eighty-five, exercise can build muscle and make a difference.

People suffering from Alzheimer's disease can and do benefit from physical therapy. The symptoms of Alzheimer's include gradual memory loss, loss of language skills, and confusion. PTs learn how to communicate with their patients who have Alzheimer's by using more gestures and gentle guidance, by learning about their patients' lives, and by validating their emotions.

As the population ages and more people live longer, physical therapy will play a major role in health care. PTs are valued by elderly people because of their skills and their ability to listen, care, and treat people as individuals.

Women's Health

PT Magazine, which is published by the APTA, notes in its June 2000 issue that during the 1990s, women's health issues finally began to get proper attention and funding. Physical therapists have expanded their role in helping women cope with special health concerns such as pelvic floor dysfunction, osteoporosis, postoperative management of mastectomy and abdominal surgery, prenatal and postdelivery dysfunction and conditioning, fibromyalgia, and injuries specific to the female athlete.

Susan Dunn, who runs the women's center within a physical therapy clinic in Kentucky and who is quoted in the *PT Magazine* article, says that she does a lot of community education programs, as well as treat patients.

> It is my mission to empower women with knowledge. I want them to know that they do not have to just suffer with conditions that "come with the territory." I want them to know what their health care options are. And I want them to feel comfortable asking their physicians for a referral to physical therapy.

Holistic Practitioners

Jan Price owns her own business in New York City, and it has two different branches. In her physical therapy practice, she treats mostly musculoskeletal injuries; she also runs a center for holistic health, where the emphasis is on prevention and wellness, and where Jan offers treatments that are not within the realm of conventional physical therapy and, in many cases, are not covered by insurance.

Many of the patients who come to Jan pay out of their own pockets. Jan works with the energy of the body and says, "There isn't a word for what I do. I call myself a PT because I am a licensed physical therapist, but holistic practitioner would be a more appropriate name." Jan is a manual therapist and also works with energy techniques.

Jan is currently studying Chinese medicine and acupuncture. Through her holistic center, she offers classes in the Feldenkrais technique, which is a well-respected method of mind-body learning. Jan is an explorer, interested in the many ways in which she can restore, maintain, and even enhance her patients' wellness, nipping health problems in the bud before they become serious, chronic conditions.

Teaching and Research

Some PTs may hold part-time or full-time teaching positions at colleges and universities. Research is another career opportunity within physical therapy. In a way, treating each patient is like doing research. For instance, even though a PT's education and training are rigorous, it is the daily experience of working with people and seeing what works and what doesn't that really builds professional knowledge and skill.

In addition to personal, everyday research, there is much formal research in the field. Several professional organizations fund and publish the results of such research. At some point, practitioners may even decide to go back to school to get an advanced degree in a field such as physical therapy, biomechanics, physiology, kinesiology, health care management, or even adult education.

Many physical therapists receive certification in a specialty and devote themselves to practice and research in such areas as pediatrics, sports medicine, or geriatrics.

A Career with Many Options

Perhaps one of the best things about a career in physical therapy is that there are so many ways to practice it. Tracy Sawyer says, "I love what I do. A lot of my friends decided that once they had a family, that's what they were going to do full-time. I could never do that. I find what I do too interesting, too exciting to stop doing it."

Margaret Plack, who has worked in a school and in a hospital, who has been in private practice, and who now heads up the PT program at Touro College, concludes:

> Sometimes you go into a field, and you're sort of narrowed by the field itself. But in physical therapy, if perchance you find that "Oh, I thought I wanted to work in pediatrics but I really don't like it," then you can go and work in a rehab center, at a nursing home, or in a clinic, or teach. It's a great profession. I absolutely love it. I wouldn't do anything different. There's not one component of physical therapy that I've tried that I've not loved, and there are still more to try.

At the core of all jobs within the field of physical therapy is a problem-solving partnership with the patient. If you are to reduce a person's physical pain, improve his or her functioning, and teach healthier and more efficient ways of moving, you must treat that person with respect and care to win trust. After all, the individuals you will be working with are letting you help them on a very intimate level—they will be including you in their efforts to improve the functioning of their bodies.

The Market for PTs and PTAs

In the 1980s, there weren't enough trained PTAs and PTs available, so they were in great demand and salaries went way up. By 2000, the field was not as "hot" as it was hyped up to be in the '80s, when many journalists wrote that there was big money to be made in physical therapy. There was some truth to that, but suddenly, some people actually started going into physical therapy for the money! If you've been reading this book, you know what a bad idea that is. Physical therapy can earn you a good living, but you have to really want to do it. Otherwise, why study so hard and give so much of yourself to your patients, day in and day out?

Today, the job market is a bit tighter. Margaret Plack says that in the early '90s, her students each had three, four, or five places that wanted to hire them. Today, her students still get good jobs, but they may not get "the pick of the litter." One of the reasons for this is simply that there are a lot more degree programs training a lot more people. Simply put, there's more competition. Also, by the end of the 1990s, insurance companies were stricter in their payments, or reimbursements, and the Balanced Budget Act of 1997 had limited funding for health care through Medicare and Medicaid.

Several of the PTs interviewed for this book make the point that although you certainly can make good money as a PT, money should not be the reason you enter the profession. You've got to want it; you've got to care. It's not easy to pinpoint exactly why salaries rise and fall and professions heat up and cool down, but the U.S. government predicts that demand for qualified PTs and PTAs will continue to increase in the twenty-first century. If you love the work, if you're suited to it and you receive a high-quality education, you will make a good living and have a meaningful, rewarding career.

Glossary

anatomy Study of the bodily structure of a human being (or animal).

assistive devices Devices that aid mobility and movement, for instance, canes, walkers, and wheelchairs.

cardiac Of or relating to the heart.

chronic Lasting over a long period of time, like certain illnesses.

clinical affiliation A physical therapy student's practical work at a health care facility; part of the student's education.

complementary therapies Techniques, sometimes drawn from alternative medicine or other disciplines, used by PTs in combination with regular physical therapy to enhance and complete treatment.

direct access Ability of a patient to go directly to a PT without first being referred by a physician.

disability Physical or mental impairment that prevents or restricts normal achievement or activity.

ergonomics Science and practice that seeks to minimize workers' fatigue, discomfort, and injury on the job.

evaluation Process whereby a PT comes to an understanding of what a patient's problem is; the first step toward healing.

fibromyalgia A condition that causes pain and stiffness in the muscles, joints, ligaments, tendons, or tissues.

function Ability of a person to do what he or she needs and/or wants to do.

geriatrics Branch of medicine that deals with the diseases and health problem of the aged.

inpatients Patients who are admitted to a hospital for treatment that requires at least one overnight stay.

kinesiology Study of the muscles and the mechanics of human motion.

manual therapy Hands-on techniques used by PTs to move, adjust, and help the body to heal.

modalities Appliances PTs use to decrease pain and build strength and flexibility.

neurology Medical science that deals with the nervous system, and diseases and conditions that affect it.

orthopedics Branch of medicine that deals with the prevention or correction of injuries or disorders of the musculoskeletal system, including the bones, muscles, joints, ligaments, and tendons.

orthotics Science that deals with the use of specialized mechanical devices to support or supplement weakened or abnormal joints or limbs; a brace is an orthotic.

outpatients Patients who are admitted to a hospital or clinic for treatment that does not require an overnight stay.

pediatrics Branch of medicine that deals with the care of infants and children and the treatment of their diseases.

physiatrist Medical doctor who is a specialist in rehabilitation and physical medicine.

physiology Biological study of the functions of the systems of the human body (or other living organisms).

prosthesis Artificial device used to replace a missing body part, such as an arm or leg.

pulmonary Of, relating to, or affecting the lungs.

range of motion (ROM) How fully a joint can allow a limb to move and bend.

referral Sending a patient to a health care provider who has a different specialty; a physician may refer a patient to a PT, and a PT may refer a patient to a physician.

rehabilitation Therapeutic process of restoring someone to good health or a useful life.

stroke Sudden loss of brain function caused by a blockage or rupture of a blood vessel in the brain; often results in paralysis or other loss of function.

therapeutic exercise Exercise that is prescribed to an individual for healing injuries or disease, or as a preventive measure.

For More Information

In the United States

American Academy of Orthopaedic Manual
 Physical Therapists (AAOMPT)
P.O. Box 4777
Biloxi, MS 39535-4777
(228) 392-0028
Web site: http://www.aaompt.org

American Association for Respiratory Care (AARC)
11030 Ables Lane
Dallas, TX 75229-4593
(972) 243-2272
Web site: http://www.aarc.org

American Physical Therapy Association (APTA)
1111 North Fairfax Street
Alexandria, VA 22314-1488
(800) 999-APTA (2782)
Web site: http://www. apta.org

American Sports Medicine Institute
Sports Medicine Camp
1313 13th Street South
Birmingham, AL 35205
(205) 918-2131
Web site: http://www.asmi.org/asmiweb/education/
   sportcamp.htm

Marquette University
Physical Therapy Program
P.O. Box 1881
Milwaukee, WI 53201-1881
(800) 222-6544
Web site: http://www.mu.edu/chs/pt/about.html

In Canada

Canadian Physiotherapy Association (CPA)
2345 Yonge Street, Suite 410
Toronto, ON M4P 2E5
(416) 932-1888
(800) 387-8679
Web site: http://www.physiotherapy.ca
CPA National Student Assembly page:
http://www.physiotherapy.ca/natstudent.htm

Web Sites

American Academy of Physical Medicine and Rehabilitation
http://www.aapmr.org

American College of Sports Medicine
http://www.acsm.org

Careers in Physical Therapy

American Medical Association
http://www.ama-assn.org

The Federation of State Boards of Physical Therapy
http://www.fsbpt.org

Geriatrics Section, American Physical Therapy Association
http://geriatricspt.org

Manual Therapy Online
http://swodeam.com/mto.html

Neurology Section, American Physical Therapy Association
http://www.neuropt.org

Nicholas Institute of Sports Medicine and Athletic Trauma
http://www.nismat.org

Physical Therapy Page at About.com
http://physicaltherapy.about.com

PTCentral
http://www.ptcentral.com

RehabEdge
http://www.rehabedge.com

Rehabilitation Institute of Chicago
http://www.rehabchicago.org

Rusk Institute of Rehabilitation Medicine
http://www.msnyuhealth.org/hso/hosp_index.jsp?hosp=ri

United States Army Physical Therapy Specialty Course
http://www.cs.amedd.army.mil/ptsc/default.htm

For Further Reading

Applegate, Edith J. *The Anatomy and Physiology Learning System*. 2nd ed. Philadelphia: W. B. Saunders, 2000.

Davis, Carol M. *Patient Practitioner Interaction: An Experiential Manual for Developing the Art of Health Care*. 3rd ed. Thorofare, NJ: Slack, 1998.

Jensen, Gail M., Jan Gwyer, Laurita M. Hack, and Katherine F. Shephard. *Expertise in Physical Therapy Practice*. Boston: Butterworth-Heinemann Medical, 1999.

Jones, Kim, and Karen Barker. *Human Movement Explained*. Boston: Butterworth-Heinemann Medical, 1996.

Krumhansl, Bernice R., and Kathy Siebel. *Opportunities in Physical Therapy Careers*. Rev. ed. Lincolnwood, IL: VGM Career Horizons, 2000.

Moffat, Marilyn, and Steve Vickery. *American Physical Therapy Association Book of Body Maintenance and Repair*. New York: Henry Holt & Company, 1999.

Morse, Gary A. *Therapist as Supervisor and Coach*. Boston: Butterworth-Heinemann Medical, 1998.

Pagliarulo, Michael A. *Introduction to Physical Therapy*. 2nd ed. St. Louis, MO: Mosby-Year Book, Inc., 2001.

Index

About the Author

Trisha Hawkins is a writer and copy editor who lives in Brooklyn, New York. She is a graduate of Harvard College.

Acknowledgments

Many thanks to the wonderful PTs and PTAs who provided information for this book: Alex Bagley, Chris Barrett, Beebe Haniff, Sue Kempner, Margaret Plack, Tracy Sawyer, Tim Tyler, Pat Walaszek, Eric Quan, and Gabriel Yankowitz. Special thanks to Joan Edelstein. Also, thanks to the American Physical Therapy Association, the Canadian Physiotherapy Association, and the New York Physical Therapy Association.

Series Design

Danielle Goldblatt

Layout

Thomas Forget